# YOUR KNOWLEDGE HAS VALUE

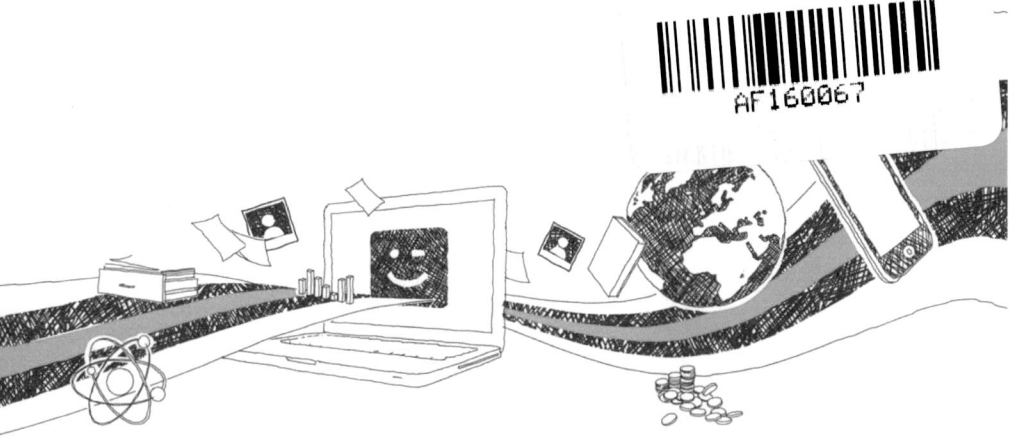

- We will publish your bachelor's and master's thesis, essays and papers

- Your own eBook and book - sold worldwide in all relevant shops

- Earn money with each sale

Upload your text at www.GRIN.com
and publish for free

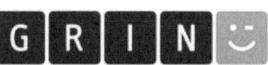

**Bibliographic information published by the German National Library:**

The German National Library lists this publication in the National Bibliography; detailed bibliographic data are available on the Internet at http://dnb.dnb.de .

This book is copyright material and must not be copied, reproduced, transferred, distributed, leased, licensed or publicly performed or used in any way except as specifically permitted in writing by the publishers, as allowed under the terms and conditions under which it was purchased or as strictly permitted by applicable copyright law. Any unauthorized distribution or use of this text may be a direct infringement of the author s and publisher s rights and those responsible may be liable in law accordingly.

**Imprint:**

Copyright © 2018 GRIN Verlag
Print and binding: Books on Demand GmbH, Norderstedt Germany
ISBN: 9783668626355

**This book at GRIN:**

https://www.grin.com/document/387500

Patrick Kimuyu

# Ethics of Physician Assisted Suicide

GRIN Verlag

## GRIN - Your knowledge has value

Since its foundation in 1998, GRIN has specialized in publishing academic texts by students, college teachers and other academics as e-book and printed book. The website www.grin.com is an ideal platform for presenting term papers, final papers, scientific essays, dissertations and specialist books.

**Visit us on the internet:**

http://www.grin.com/

http://www.facebook.com/grincom

http://www.twitter.com/grin_com

Ethics of Physician Assisted Suicide

Name: Patrick Kimuyu

## Introduction

Physician assisted suicide has become one of the most contentious ethical issues in the United States of America. The current debate over whether euthanasia (physician-assisted suicide) should be legalized or not has evoked unprecedented controversy in the society because in this practice seems to encompass some ethical problems. Interestingly, physician-assisted suicide seem to have been used as a useful medical approach over a long time, even before the emergence of the controversial debate that seems to be assuming divergent directions day-by-day. It is also amusing to learn that those who are involved in the physician-assisted debate are not the beneficiaries of the practice. Initially, the precepts of the physician-assisted suicide imply that a terminally ill individual can request for a painless termination of his or her life, solely out of the individual's wishes (Welie & Ten-Have, 2005). In addition, relatives to the ailing individual can request for the termination of the life of their loved one to avoid unnecessary agony and suffering. Moreover, the decision to terminate the life of a terminally ill individual can be made by the physicians depending with the severity of the disease condition. All these precepts agree with the terms of euthanasia, which defines it as "easy death" according to the Greeks who called it *euthanatos* (Keown, 2002). Physician-assisted suicide issue has turned out to be an ethical dilemma among the U.S population because; there is no universal explanation which is provided by the popularly known normative theories. These theories address the issue of physician-assisted suicide from diverse perspectives, leading to the observed ethical conflict. The other aspect of the physician-assisted suicide lies within the medical ethics. Physicians seem to be tied up by the medical ethics especially through the Hippocratic Oath, and yet they are ought to facilitate the practice. Therefore, this critical paper discusses euthanasia and its ethics.

## Ethics of Physician Assisted Suicide

In general, the principal ethical issue that has evoked the debate over the physician-assisted suicide is the rhetoric nature of the three key ethical questions that seek to tone down the ambiguous aspect of the practice. It is obvious that the current debate over the issue of physician-assisted suicide is not necessarily about legalization, but rather about the ethical questions whose answers remain uncertain. These questions seek to define some of the cultural aspects and societal norms especially among the U.S population.

From an ethical perspective, the debate about the physician-assisted suicide comprises of questions that attempt to establish a universal conclusion over the issue, despite the ambiguity created by the current normative theories. The question, "Is it right to terminate one's life?" seeks for the answer whether the physician-assisted suicide conforms to the societal norms and values. Ordinarily, suicide is regarded to as a social vice in the society. Therefore, physician-assisted suicide is usually considered to be an intended violation of the social norms of the society. In contrast, this practice has been incorporated into the current medical approaches and its application as a reliable tool is seemingly gaining unprecedented popularity.

In addition, the second question, "Is it ethical for someone to help a terminally ill individual to die?" seeks to get a validation of the physicians' role in helping the terminally ill individuals to undergo a painless death (Welie & Ten-Have, 2005). This question appears to be the most contentious ethical issue because; it poses a significant challenge to the Hippocratic Oath that requires physicians to protect the patient's life at all cost. From a retrospective perspective, the Hippocratic Oath forbids physicians from facilitating for the death of the patient; instead, they are supposed to employ relentless efforts to keep the patient alive. Therefore, physician-assisted suicide places the physician at the central point of the matter, and this appears to compromise the professional code of ethics. As a result, physicians are pushed into the Island of controversy because they cannot validate their role. According to the Hippocratic Oath, it is wrong for a physician to contribute in any way to the death of the patient. In contrast, euthanasia has been adopted as one of the reliable medical approaches that help patients to avoid unbearable pain.

On the other hand, the question, "Is it right to kill others upon their own request to be killed?" attempts to validate an individual's right to make critical choices over their lives, especially with matters related to life and death (Welie & Ten-Have, 2005). It also seeks to establish a universal justification over whether other people have the right to make decisions over the lives of others. This is because; family members have been granted an opportunity to request for the termination of the life of their beloved ones depending with the ethical issues created by the patient's illness. Moreover, this question seeks for a reliable explanation of the most fundamental phenomena of mankind. It appears engrossing that human beings do not decide to be born, and the laws of nature demands that death should be unintentional, but rather a natural phenomenon. Therefore, it seems that no one has the right to decide whether to live or die.

Physician-assisted suicide seems to encompass several ethical problems, although most of them are depended on the form of euthanasia. Initially, practice of physician-assisted suicide was introduced in the medical field as a result of advancements in medicine and technology. This prompted the social change of the western culture, leading to unprecedented change in the meaning of death. Unfortunately, technological advancements in the field of medicine did not incorporate some of the fundamental ethics of the western culture.

One of the most potential harms of the physician-assisted suicide is that, it may be executed without the consent of the terminally ill individual. For instance, in involuntary euthanasia, other parties such as family members request for the termination of one's life and such decision may go against the wishes of the subject. This is a critical, ethical problem that may evoke numerous social abnormalities in the society, in case efficient guidelines are formulated to define the circumstances upon which people, rather than, the subject can request for the termination of the life of their family member who faces untreatable health condition. It appears that granting family members an opportunity to request for the termination of the life of one of their family members may allow innocent individuals to be killed against their wishes, leading to the emergence of adverse moral consequences.

Secondly, allowing physician-assisted suicide may enable relatives of the subject to perpetuate their own interests that go against the wishes of the ailing individual. For instance, people can request for the killing of their family member for their own benefit and not necessarily for the benefits of the subject. As a result, innocent individuals may be subjected to untimely death, owing to the wishes of the relatives. It appears quite shocking to imagine that an innocent individual is taken to the hospital for the termination of his or her life without the subject's request. It is extremely dehumanizing because such a circumstance may arouse immense societal outcry especially when the killed individual opposed the decision of physician-assisted suicide.

Thirdly, physician-assisted suicide appears to encompass the problem of uncertainty of the core reasons that may require family members to request for the termination of the lives of their beloved ones. It is seemingly true that, allowing relatives to request for the termination of the lives of their ailing members may prompt for the killing of innocent individuals on other reasons rather than relieving them of pain and agony. For instance, relatives who express hatred upon their family members may request for the termination of their lives without the consent of the involved subjects.

In general, physician-assisted suicide practice evokes ethical problems that seem to impart moral consequences into the issue. The current ethical problems have been occasioned by the cultural change among the western population over the last century, owing to the impacts of modernity and civilization.

From an ethical perspective, the problems that are associated to the physician-assisted suicide can be solved by the Utilitarian theory because it defines the fundamental aspects of utility. Utilitarian theory addresses all the moral aspects that touch religious beliefs and the general moral aspects of human life. According to the utilitarianism, utility refers to any moral aspect that concerns the well-being of sentient beings. Therefore, it puts into consideration all moral issues that contribute to pleasure in life. It also addresses other physical aspects such as the absence of pain. In general, the utilitarianism theory will ensure that the suicide decision will follow the most appropriate philosophical approach. According to Hooker "It shall also follow conventional philosophical opinion in supposing that it is possible to be in such a bad condition that death would be a welcome release"(Hooker. n.d, p. 23). This theory states that physician-assisted suicide serves as a reliable alternative of avoiding pain and agony. Moreover, utilitarians hold that the religious beliefs are not entirely overlooked through terminating one's life as a result of unbearable pain.

However, there are two distinct versions of utilitarianism, although their fundamental tenets are relatively the same with regard to their moral connotations. There are also different versions within the principal utilitarian versions. Utilitarianism consists of the Act-utilitarianism and the Rule-utilitarianism versions, which attempts to explain the nature of utility primarily over moral issues. Act-utilitarianism justifies the patient's decision of requesting for physician-assisted suicide. One of the versions of the Act-utilitarianism explains the actual consequences that necessitate physician-assisted suicide, while another version explains the degree of utility that justify physician-assisted suicide.

The tenets of the Act-utilitarianism holds that, "…an act is right if and only if its actual consequences would contain at least as much utility as those of any other act open to the agent" (Hooker, n.d, p. 24). Therefore, physician-assisted suicide holds greater utility than any other form of death because it helps to relieve the patient of extreme pain and agony that are caused by the disease condition. Another version of the Act-utilitarianism holds that, "…an act is right if and only if its expected utility is at least as great as that of any alternative" (Hooker, n.d, p. 24). The latter seems to support physician-assisted suicide through stating that an act is right, as long as, its expected utility carries substantial significance as any other alternative. In the case of physician-assisted suicide, putting a terminally ill individual to death is as great as relieving that individual of extreme pain through medical treatment.

On the other hand, the Rule-utilitarianism seems to differ significantly from the Act-utilitarianism in that, it does not evaluate the acts solely by their degree of utility; instead, the Rule-utilitarianism justifies any act depending with a set of conventional rules (Hinman, 2010). According to the Rule-utilitarianism, the rules followed to justify an act are determined by the terms of their accrued utility. In general, the Rule-utilitarianism holds, "…an act is morally permissible if and only if the rules with the greatest expected utility would allow it" (Hooker, n.d, p. 24). The precepts of this version of the Rule-utilitarianism hold that the expected utilities of rules are based on the majority opinion. Therefore, the Rule-utilitarianism version justifies the physician's role in executing physician-assisted suicide because it requires one to internalize the concerned rule. They will be able to decide whether to follow their consciousness and empathy in relieving the patient of unnecessary agony; rather than upholding the tenets of the Hippocratic Oath that compels physicians to protect the lives of their patients at all cost.

In contrast to the Utilitarianism theory that justifies acts by their utility, the Emotivism theory defines ethical statements according to an individual's personal understanding and choice; hence it regards them as meaningless (Vlach, n.d). This theory seems to justify physician-assisted suicide through associating death with dignity. It holds that moral statements are either true or false depending with one's overall feeling about the concerned ethical issues. Therefore, it allows all the concerned parties to make decisions on their own without influence from other peoples' opinions. For instance, the Emotivism theory justifies the patient's decision to request for physician-assisted suicide because the patient views the issue from his or her own perspective. On the other hand, it provides physicians with unchallenged opportunity of making decisions over their patients where necessary. Moreover, this theory downplays any unwarranted criticism that may arise over the issue of physician-assisted suicide because it gives all parties freedom to follow their consciousness in decision-making, especially with regard to matters related to life and death.

From a personal point of view, the utilitarianism theory seems to provide a conventional approach of understanding physician-assisted suicide, and it justifies the use of the practice as a fundamental medical approach. It also attempts to address the key ethical problems because it justifies the act of suicide according to its utility and terms of conventionally defined rules. It appears that the utilitarianism theory is the most appropriate normative theory that can solve the issue of euthanasia because it incorporates all aspects of morality, including religious beliefs.

Emotivism theory does not encompass the element of conventional understanding because an individual justify their acts according to their feelings, but not in accordance to the eternal verities of life.

## Conclusion

In a brief conclusion, physician-assisted suicide seems to have elicited unprecedented ethical issues that seem to compromise its legalization. The practice has been criticized by various groups of individuals, while others are in full support of it, especially the medical professionals. Utilitarians support the practice because they believe that physician-assisted suicide leaves the ailing patients with freedom of making decisions over their lives. In contrast, the Emotivism theory provides an opportunity for the incorporation of harmful decisions because it requires someone to follow his or her feelings.

## References

Hinman, L. (2010). *Utilitarianism*. Retrieved from

http://www.ethicsmatters.net/presentations/socialethics/Theory/Utilitarianism.pdf

Hooker, B. (n.d). *Rule-Utilitarianism and Euthanasia*. Retrieved from

http://www.blackwellpublishing.com/content/BPL_Images/Content_store/Sample_chapter/9780631228332/lafollette.pdf

Keown, J. (2002). *Euthanasia, Ethics and Public Policy: An Argument against Legalisation*. Cambridge, UK: Cambridge University Press. Retrieved from

http://assets.cambridge.org/97805218/04165/sample/9780521804165ws.pdf

Vlach, M. (n.d). *Emotivism*. Retrieved from http://www.theologicalstudies.org/resource-library/philosophy-dictionary/110-emotivism

Welie, J. & Ten-Have, A. (2005). *Death and Medical Power: An Ethical Analysis of Dutch Euthanasia Practice*. Maidenhead, England: Open University Press.

# YOUR KNOWLEDGE HAS VALUE

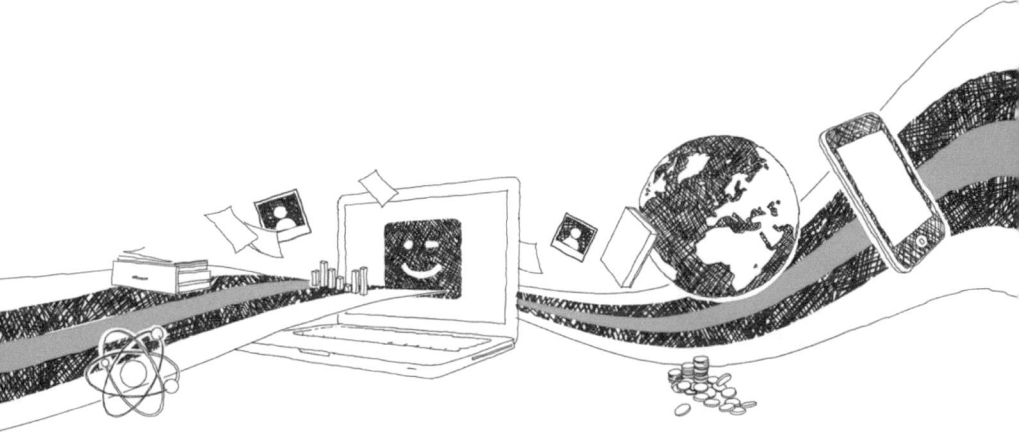

- We will publish your bachelor's and master's thesis, essays and papers

- Your own eBook and book - sold worldwide in all relevant shops

- Earn money with each sale

Upload your text at www.GRIN.com
and publish for free

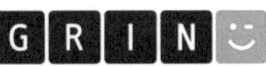